Keto Diet Cookbook

Easy Keto Recipes to Lose Weight and Boost Metabolism while Satisfying your Cravings

Claudia Giordano

© **Copyright 2021 - All rights reserved.**

The content contained within this book may not be reproduced, duplicated or transmitted without direct written permission from the author or the publisher.

Under no circumstances will any blame or legal responsibility be held against the publisher, or author, for any damages, reparation, or monetary loss due to the information contained within this book. Either directly or indirectly.

Legal Notice:

This book is copyright protected. This book is only for personal use. You cannot amend, distribute, sell, use, quote or paraphrase any part, or the content within this book, without the consent of the author or publisher.

Disclaimer Notice:

Please note the information contained within this document is for educational and entertainment purposes only. All effort has been executed to present accurate, up to date, and reliable, complete information. No warranties of any kind are declared or implied. Readers acknowledge that the author is not engaging in the rendering of legal, financial, medical or professional advice. The content within this book has been derived from various sources. Please consult a licensed professional before attempting any techniques outlined in this book.

By reading this document, the reader agrees that under no circumstances is the author responsible for any losses, direct or indirect, which are incurred as a result of the use of information contained within this document, including, but not limited to, errors, omissions, or inaccuracies.

Ketogenic Diet For Beginners

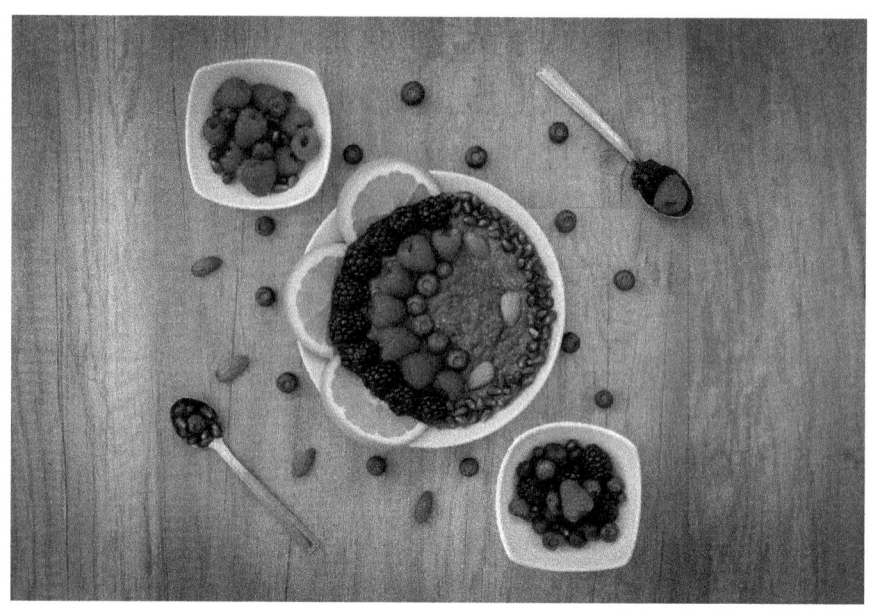

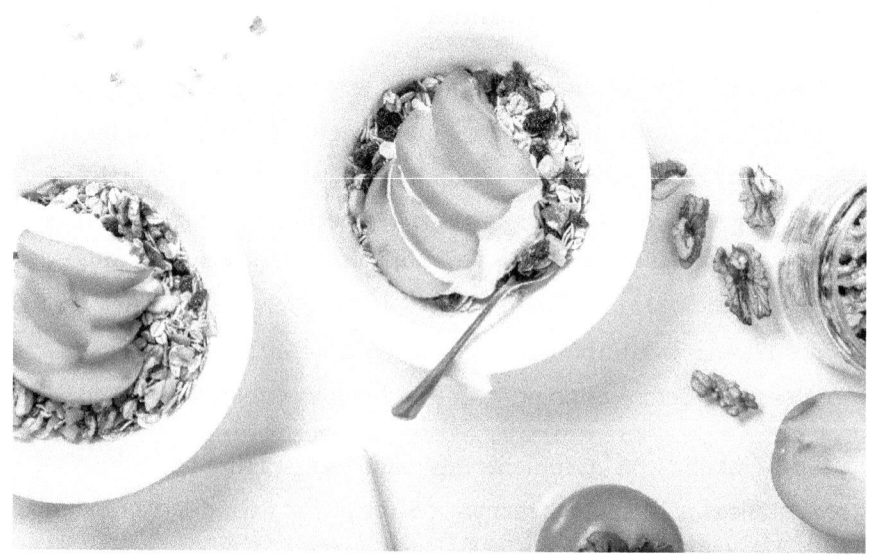

Table of contents

WHAT IS A KETO DIET? **8**
KETOGENIC RECIPES FOR BREAKFAST **12**
    1. Chili Tomatoes And Eggs 12
    2. Mushroom Omelet 14
    3. Bell Peppers and Avocado Bowls 16
    4. Spinach and Eggs Salad 18
    5. Creamy Eggs 20
    6. Shrimp and Eggs Mix 22

KETOGENIC RECIPES FOR LUNCH **24**
    7. Turkey Salad 24
    8. Cheesy Turkey Pan 26
    9. Chicken and Leeks Pan 28
    10. Chicken and Peppers Mix 30

KETOGENIC SIDE DISH RECIPES **32**
    11. Cabbage Saute 32
    12. Paprika Napa Cabbage 34
    13. Cauliflower and Radish Mix 36
    14. Basil Zucchini and Tomatoes 38
    15. Sesame Green Beans 40
    16. Green Beans and Pine Nuts Mix 42

KETOGENIC SNACKS AND APPETIZERS RECIPES **44**
    17. Herbed Cheese Dip 44
    18. Cheesy Beef Dip 46
    19. Broccoli Dip 48
    20. Pesto Dip 50
    21. Zucchini Muffins 51

KETOGENIC FISH AND SEAFOOD RECIPES **54**
    22. Creamy Mackerel 54

- 23. LIME MACKEREL 56
- 24. TURMERIC TILAPIA 58
- 25. WALNUT SALMON MIX 60
- 26. CHIVES TROUT 62
- 27. SALMON AND TOMATOES 64

KETOGENIC POULTRY RECIPES 66

- 28. GHEE CHICKEN MIX 66
- 29. PAPRIKA CHICKEN WINGS 68
- 30. CHICKEN AND CAPERS 70
- 31. CILANTRO WINGS 72
- 32. BAKED TURKEY MIX 74
- 33. TURKEY AND ARTICHOKES MIX 76

KETOGENICMEATRECIPES 78

- 34. PORK AND TOMATOES 78
- 35. GARLIC PORK AND ZUCCHINIS 80
- 36. BALSAMIC PORK CHOPS 82
- 37. ROSEMARY PORK 84

KETOGENICVEGETABLERECIPES 86

- 38. BROCCOLI CREAM 86
- 39. BAKED BROCCOLI 88

KETOGENIC DESSERT RECIPES 90

- 40. CHOCOLATE PUDDING 90

Ketogenic Diet For Beginners

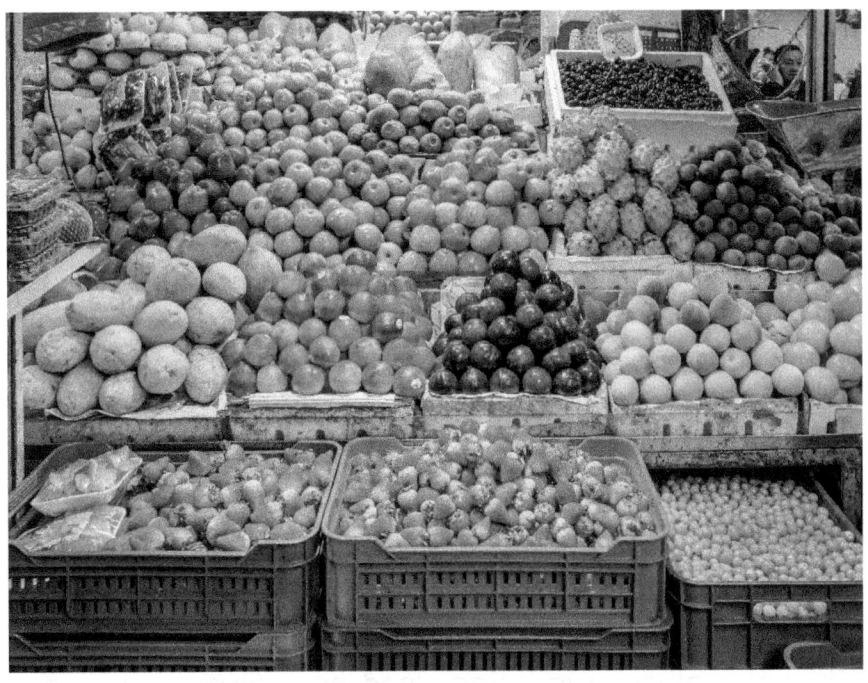

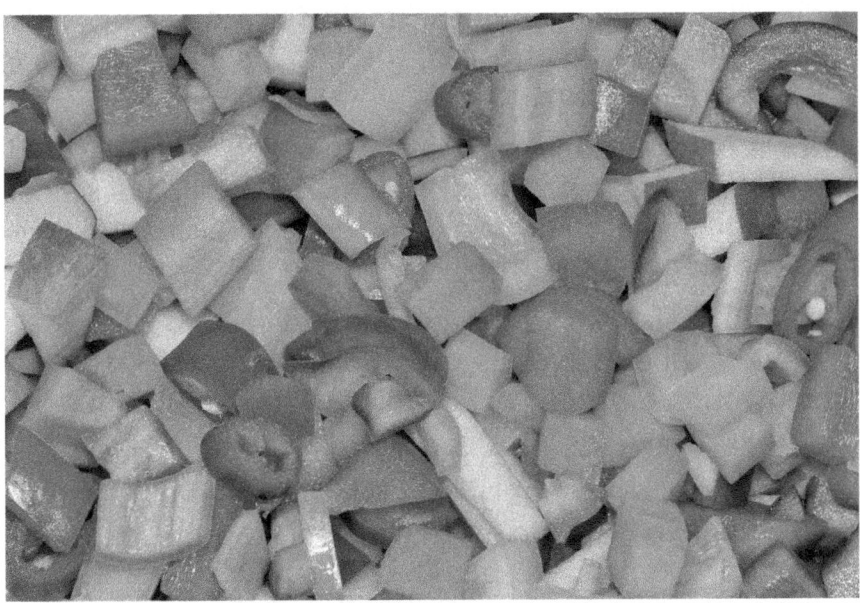

WHAT IS A KETO DiET?

A keto diet is well known for being a low carb diet, where the body produces ketones in the liver to be used as energy. It's referred to as many different names – ketogenic diet, low carb diet, low carb high fat (LCHF), etc.

When you eat something high in carbs, your body will produce glucose and insulin.

Glucose is the easiest molecule for your body to convert and use as energy so that it will be chosen over any other energy source.

Insulin is produced to process the glucose in your bloodstream by taking it around the body.

Since the glucose is being used as a primary energy, your fats are not needed and are therefore stored. Typically on a normal, higher carbohydrate diet, the body will use glucose as the main form of energy. By lowering the intake of carbs, the body is induced into a state known as ketosis.

Ketosis is a natural process the body initiates to help us survive when food intake is low. During this state, we produce ketones, which are produced from the breakdown of fats in the liver.

The end goal of a properly maintained keto diet is to force your body into this metabolic state. We don't do this through starvation of calories but starvation of carbohydrates.

Our bodies are incredibly adaptive to what you put into it – when you overload it with fats and take away carbohydrates, it will begin to burn ketones as the primary energy source. Optimal ketone levels offer many health, weight loss, physical and mental performance benefits.

Benefits of a Ketogenic Diet

There are numerous benefits that come with being on keto: from weight loss and increased energy levels to therapeutic medical applications. Most anyone can safely benefit from eating a low-carb, high-fat diet.

Weight Loss

The ketogenic diet essentially uses your body fat as an energy source – so there are obvious weight loss benefits. On keto, your insulin (the fat storing hormone) levels drop greatly which turns your body into a fat burning machine.

Scientifically, the ketogenic diet has shown better results compared to low-fat and high- carb diets; even in the long term.

Many people incorporate MCT Oil into their diet (it increases ketone production and fat loss) by drinking bulletproof coffee in the morning.

Control Blood Sugar

Keto naturally lowers blood sugar levels due to the type of foods you eat. Studies even show that the ketogenic diet is a more effective way to manage and prevent diabetes compared to low-calorie diets

If you're pre-diabetic or have Type II diabetes, you should seriously consider a ketogenic diet. We have many readers that have had success with their blood sugar control on keto.

Mental Focus

Many people use the ketogenic diet specifically for the increased mental performance.

Ketones are a great source of fuel for the brain. When you lower carb intake, you avoid big spikes in blood sugar. Together, this can result in improved focus and concentration.

Studies show that an increased intake of fatty acids can have impacting benefits to our brain's function.

Increased Energy & Normalized Hunger

By giving your body a better and more reliable energy source, you will feel more energized during the day. Fats are shown to be the most effective molecule to burn as fuel.

On top of that, fat is naturally more satisfying and ends up leaving us in a satiated ("full") state for longer.

Epilepsy

The ketogenic diet has been used since the early 1900's to treat epilepsy successfully. It is still one of the most widely used therapies for children who have uncontrolled epilepsy today.

One of the main benefits of the ketogenic diet and epilepsy is that it allows fewer medications to be used while still offering excellent control.

In the last few years, studies have also shown significant results in adults treated with keto as well.

Cholesterol & Blood Pressure

A keto diet has shown to improve triglyceride levels and cholesterol levels most associated with arterial buildup. More specifically low-carb, high-fat diets show a dramatic increase in HDL and decrease in LDL particle concentration compared to low-fat diets.

Many studies on low-carb diets show better improvement in blood pressure over other diets.

Some blood pressure issues are associated with excess weight, which is a bonus since keto tends to lead to weight loss.

Insulin Resistance

Insulin resistance can lead to type II diabetes if left unmanaged. An abundant amount of research shows that a low carb, ketogenic diet can help people lower their insulin levels to healthy ranges.

Even if you're athletic, you can benefit from insulin optimization on keto through eating foods high in omega-3 fatty acids.

Acne

It's common to experience improvements in your skin when you switch to a ketogenic diet.

For acne, it may be beneficial to reduce dairy intake and follow a strict skin cleaning regimen..

KETOGENIC RECIPES FOR BREAKFAST

1. Chili Tomatoes And Eggs

This recipe is perfect for breakfast!

Preparation time: 10 minutes

Cooking time : 20 minutes

Servings: 4

Ingredients:

- 1 tablespoon ghee, melted
- 2 shallots, chopped
- 2 chili peppers, minced
- Salt and black pepper to the taste
- 4 tomatoes, cubed
- 4 eggs, whisked

- 1 teaspoon sweet paprika
- 1 tablespoon chives, chopped

Directions:

1. Heat up a pan with the ghee over medium heat, add the shallots and the chili peppers, toss andsauté for 5 minutes.
2. Add the tomatoes and the other ingredients except the eggs, toss and cook everything for 5minutes more.
3. Add the eggs, toss a bit, cook the mix for another 5 minutes, divide between plates and serve.

Nutrition:

- Calories 119 Fat 7.9 Fiber 1.8
- Carbs 6.5
- Protein 6.9

2. Mushroom Omelet

You will feel full of energy all day with this keto breakfast!

Preparationtime : 10 minutes

Cooking time : 20 minutes

Servings : 4

Ingredients:

- 2 spring onions, chopped
- ½ pound white mushrooms
- Salt and black pepper to the taste
- 4 eggs, whisked 1 tablespoon olive oil
- ½ teaspoon cumin, ground
- 1 tablespoon cilantro, chopped

Directions:

1. Heat up a pan with the oil over medium heat, add

the spring onions and the mushrooms, toss andsauté for 5 minutes.

2. Add the eggs and the rest of the ingredients, toss gently, spread into the pan, cover it and cookover medium heat for 15 minutes.

3. Slice the omelet, divide it between plates and serve for breakfast.

Nutrition:

- Calories 109,
- Fat 8.1,
- Fiber 0.8,
- Carbs 2.9
- Protein 7.5

3. Bell Peppers and Avocado Bowls

Try a different keto breakfast each day!

Preparation time: 10 minutes

Cooking time: 15 minutes

Servings: 4

Ingredients:

- 2 tablespoons olive oil
- 2 shallots, chopped
- 1 red bell pepper, cut into strips
- 1 yellow bell pepper, cut into strips
- 1 green bell pepper, cut into strips
- 1 big avocado, peeled, pitted and cut into wedges
- 1 teaspoon sweet paprika
- ½ cup vegetable stock
- Salt and black pepper to the taste
- 1 tablespoon chives, chopped

Directions:

1. Heat up a pan with the oil medium heat, add the shallots and sauté them for 2 minutes.
2. Add the bell peppers, avocado and the other ingredients except the chives, toss, bring to asimmer and cook over medium heat for 13 minutes more.
3. Add the chives, toss, divide into bowls and serve for breakfast.

Nutrition:

- Calories 194
- Fat 17.1
- Fiber 4.9
- Carbs 11.5
- Protein 2

4. Spinach and Eggs Salad

This taste delicious!

Preparation time: 5 minutes

Cooking time: 0 minutes

Servings: 4

Ingredients:

- 2 cups baby spinach
- 1 cup cherry tomatoes, cubed
- 1 tablespoon chives, chopped
- 4 eggs, hard boiled, peeled and roughly cubed
- Salt and black pepper to the taste
- 1 tablespoon lime juice
- 1 tablespoon olive oil

Directions:

1. In a bowl, combine the spinach with the

tomatoes and the other ingredients, toss and serve forbreakfast right away.

Nutrition:

- Calories 107
- Fat 8
- Fiber 0.9
- Carbs 3.6
- Protein 6.4

5. Creamy Eggs

It's so tasty!

Preparation time: 10 minutes

Cooking time: 15 minutes

Servings: 4

Ingredients:

- 8 eggs, whisked 2 spring onions, chopped
- 1 tablespoon olive oil
- ½ cup heavy cream
- Salt and black pepper to the taste
- ½ cup mozzarella, shredded
- 1 tablespoon chives, chopped

Directions:

1. Heat up a pan with the oil over medium heat, add the spring onions, toss and sauté them for

3minutes.

2. Add the eggs mixed with the cream, salt and pepper and stir into the pan.
3. Sprinkle the mozzarella, on top, cook the mix for 12 minutes, divide it between plates, sprinklethe chives on top and serve.

Nutrition:

- Calories 220
- Fat 18.5
- Fiber 0.2
- Carbs 1.8
- Protein 12.5

6. Shrimp and Eggs Mix

It will surprise you with its taste!

Preparation time: 5 minutes

Cooking time: 11 minutes

Servings: 4

Ingredients:

- 8 eggs, whisked
- 1 tablespoon olive oil
- ½ pound shrimp, peeled, deveined and roughly chopped ¼ cup green onions, chopped
- 1 teaspoon sweet paprika
- Salt and black pepper to the taste
- 1 tablespoon cilantro, chopped

Directions:

1. Heat up a pan with the oil over medium heat, add

the spring onions, toss and sauté for 2 minutes.

2. Add the shrimp, stir and cook for 4 minutes more.
3. Add the eggs, paprika, salt and pepper, toss and cook for 5 minutes more.
4. Divide the mix between plates, sprinkle the cilantro on top and serve for breakfast.

Nutrition:

- Calories 227
- Fat 13.3
- Fiber 0.4
- Carbs 2.3
- Protein 24.2

KETOGENIC RECIPES FOR LUNCH

7. Turkey Salad

This ispackedwithhealthyelements and it's 100% keto!

Preparationtime : 5 minutes

Cooking time : 0 minutes

Servings : 4

Ingredients:

- 1 cup cherry tomatoes, halved
- 1 cucumber, sliced
- 1 carrot, grated
- Salt and black pepper to the taste
- 1 tablespoonbalsamicvinegar
- 1 tablespoon olive oil

- 1 and ½ cups turkeybreast, cooked, skinless, boneless and shredded

Directions:

1. In a salad bowl, combine the turkeywith the tomatoes, cucumber and the otheringredients, toss and serve for lunch.

Nutrition:

- Calories 57
- Fat 3.7
- Fiber 1.3
- Carbs 6.1
- Protein 1.2

8. Cheesy Turkey Pan

It's an easy and tasty lunch idea for all thosewho are on a Ketodiet!

Preparation time: 10 minutes

Cooking time: 25 minutes

Servings: 4

Ingredients:

- 2 cups cheddar cheese, grated
- 1 big turkeybreast, skinless, boneless and cubed
- 1 tablespoontomatopassata
- ¼ cup veggie stock
- 1 tablespoon olive oil
- 2 shallots, chopped
- ¼ cup tomatoes, cubed
- Salt and black pepper to the taste

Directions:

1. Heat up a pan with the oil over medium heat, add the shallots and sauté for 2minutes.
2. Add the meat and brown for 5 minutes.
3. Ad the passata and the otheringredientsexcept the cheese, toss and cookovermediumheat for 10 minutes more.
4. Sprinkle the cheese on top, cookeverything for 7-8 minutes, dividebetweenplates and serve for lunch.

Nutrition:

- Calories 309
- Fat 23.1
- Fiber 0.4
- Carbs 3.9
- Protein 21.6

9. Chicken and Leeks Pan

Werecommendyou to trythisKetogenic pizza for lunch today!

Preparation time: 10 minutes

Cooking time: 20 minutes

Servings: 4

Ingredients:

- 2 tablespoons olive oil
- 1 pound chickenbreast, skinless, boneless and cutintostrips
- 2 shallots, chopped
- 1 cup mozzarella cheese, shredded
- 2 leeks, sliced
- ½ cup veggie stock
- 1 tablespoonheavycream
- 1 teaspoonsweet paprika

- Salt and black pepper to the taste

Directions:

1. Heat up a pan with the oil over medium heat, add the shallots, stir and cook for 3minutes.
2. Add the meat and the leeks, stir and brown for 7 minutes more.
3. Add the otheringredientsexcept the cheese and stir.
4. Sprinkle the cheese on top, introduce the pan in the oven and cookeverything at400 degrees F for 10 minutes more.
5. Divide the mix between plates and serve.

Nutrition:

- Calories 253 Fat 12.9 Fiber 1
- Carbs 7.2
- Protein 26.9

10. Chicken and Peppers Mix

This tastes so divine! They are soamazing!

Preparation time: 10 minutes

Cooking time: 25 minutes

Servings: 4

Ingredients:

- 1 cup redbellpeppers, cutintostrips
- 1 pound chickenbreast, skinless, boneless and roughlycubed
- 2 springonions, chopped
- 2 tablespoons olive oil
- 1 tomato, cubed
- Salt and black pepper to the taste
- ¼ cup tomatopassata
- 1 tablespooncilantro, chopped

Directions:

1. Heat up a pan with the oil over medium heat, add the springonions and sautéthem for 2 minutes.
2. Add the chicken and the bellpeppers, stir and cookeverything for 8 minutesmore.
3. Add the rest of the ingredients, bring to a simmer and cook over medium heat for15 minutes more stirringoften.
4. Divide the mix between plates and serve

Nutrition:

- Calories 206
- Fat 10
- Fiber 0.9
- Carbs 3.7
- Protein 24.8

KETOGENIC SIDE DISH

RECIPES

11. Cabbage Sauté

Serve thiswith a steak!

Preparation time: 10 minutes

Cooking time: 15 minutes

Servings: 4

Ingredients:

- 1 big green cabbagehead, roughlyshredded
- 2 shallots, chopped
- 1 tablespoon olive oil
- ½ cup veggie stock
- ½ cup tomatopassata
- 1 tablespoondill, chopped

Directions:

1. Heat up a pan with the oil over medium heat, add the shallots and sauté for 2minutes.
2. Add the cabbage, stir and cook for 3 minutes more.
3. Add the rest of the ingredients, toss, bring to a simmer and cook over mediumheat for 10 minutes more.
4. Divide the sauté between plates and serve.

Nutrition:

- Calories 97
- Fat 4
- Fiber 6
- Carbs 15.2
- Protein 3.5

12. Paprika Napa Cabbage

You willdefinitelyenjoythisgreatsidedish!

Preparation time: 10 minutes Cooking time: 20 minutes Servings: 4

Ingredients:

- 4 cups napacabbage, roughlyshredded
- 2 tablespoonsavocadooil
- 2 springonions, chopped
- ½ teaspoongarlicpowder
- 1 teaspoonsweet paprika
- ½ cup veggie stock
- 1 tablespooncilantro, chopped

Directions:

1. Heat up a pan with the oil over medium heat, add the springonions, stirandsauté for 2 minutes.

2. Add the cabbage and the otheringredients, toss, bring to a simmer and cook for18 minutes more.
3. Divide the mix between plates and serve.

Nutrition:

- Calories 25
- Fat 1.4
- Fiber 1.5
- Carbs 3.3
- Protein 1.4

13. Cauliflower and Radish Mix

This simple Ketogenic sauté isawesome!

Preparation time: 10 minutes

Cooking time: 15 minutes Servings: 4

Ingredients:

- ¼ cup veggie stock
- 1 tablespoon olive oil
- 3 garliccloves, minced
- 1 cauliflowerhead, floretsseparated
- A pinch of salt and black pepper
- 1 cup radishes, cubed
- 2 tablespoonsrosemary, chopped

Directions:

1. Heat up a pan with the oil over medium heat, add the garlic and sauté for 2minutes.

2. Add the cauliflower and the otheringredients, toss, bring to a simmer and cookover medium heat for 13 minutes more.
3. Divide the mix between plates and serve as a sidedish.

Nutrition:

- Calories 61
- Fat 4
- Fiber 2.9
- Carbs 6.4
- Protein 1.7

14. Basil Zucchini and Tomatoes

These are simply the best! It's a greatketosidedish!

Preparation time: 10 minutes

Cooking time: 18 minutes Servings: 4

Ingredients:

- 2 zucchinis, roughlycubed
- ½ pound cherry tomatoes, halved
- 2 shallots, chopped
- 2 tablespoons olive oil
- ½ cup veggie stock
- A pinch of salt and black pepper
- 1 tablespoonbasil, chopped
- 2 tablespoonsbalsamicvinegar

Directions:

1. Heat up a pan with the oil over medium heat, add

the shallots, stir and sauté for 3minutes.

2. Add the zucchinis and the otheringredients, toss, cook over medium heat for 15minutes more, dividebetween plates and serve.

Nutrition:

- Calories 93
- Fat 7.5
- Fiber 1.8
- Carbs 6.7
- Protein 1.8

15. Sesame Green Beans

This is an amazingsidedishyou must try!

Preparation time: 10 minutes

Cooking time: 20 minutes

Servings: 4

Ingredients:

- 1 pound green beans, trimmed and halved
- 2 green onions, chopped
- 1 tablespoonavocadooil
- 2 garliccloves, minced
- 1 tablespoonbalsamicvinegar
- ½ cup chicken stock
- Salt and black pepper to the taste
- 1 teaspoonsesameseeds
- 1 tablespoondill, chopped

Directions:

1. Heat up a pan with the oil over medium high heat, add the green onionsandthegarlic, stir and sauté for 2 minutes.
2. Add the green beans and the otheringredientsexcept the sesameseeds, toss, bring to a simmer and cook over medium heat for 18 minutes.
3. Divide the mix between plates, sprinkle the sesameseeds on top and serve.

Nutrition:

- Calories 110
- Fat 4
- Fiber 4
- Carbs 6
- Protein 4

16. Green Beans and Pine Nuts Mix

This can beservedwith a chickendish!

Preparation time: 10 minutes

Cooking time: 15 minutes Servings: 4

Ingredients:

- 2 tablespoons olive oil
- 1 pound green beans, trimmed and halved
- 2 tablespoons pine nuts
- 3 garliccloves, minced
- ¼ cup parmesan cheese, grated
- 1 tablespooncilantro, chopped
- A pinch of salt and black pepper

Directions:

1. Heat up a pan with the oil over medium heat, add

the garlic and the pine nutsandcook for 5 minutes.

2. Add the green beans, and the otheringredients, toss, cook for 10 minutes more,dividebetween plates and serve as a sidedish.

Nutrition:

- Calories 100
- Fat 7
- Fiber 3
- Carbs 5.1
- Protein 5

KETOGENIC SNACKS AND APPETIZERS RECIPES

17. Herbed Cheese Dip

It's a fact! Theseisdelicious!

Preparation time: 10 minutes

Cooking time: 20 minutes Servings: 4

Ingredients:

- A pinch of salt and black pepper
- 2 shallots, chopped 6 ouncescreamcheese, soft
- 1 tablespooncilantro, chopped
- 1 tablespoonchives, chopped

Directions:

1. In a bowl combine the creamcheesewith the

shallots and the otheringredients,whisk and divideinto 4 ramekins.

2. Introduce the ramekins in the oven, cook at 380 degrees F for 20 minutes andserve as a party dip.

Nutrition:

- Calories 152
- Fat 14.9
- Fiber 0
- Carbs 2
- Protein 3.4

18. Cheesy Beef Dip

This is a great snack idea!

Preparation time: 10 minutes

Cooking time: 35 minutes Servings: 6

Ingredients:

- 8 ouncescreamcheese, soft
- A pinch of salt and black pepper
- 8 ouncesbeefstewmeat, ground
- 2 shallots, chopped
- 2 tablespoons olive oil
- ¼ cup green onions, chopped

Directions:

1. Heat up a pan with the oil over medium heat, add the shallots and the greenonions, stir and cook for 5 minutes.

2. Add the meat and brown for 5 minutes more.

3. Add the cream, salt and pepper, whisk, divideinto 6 smallramekins, introducethem in the oven and cook at 380 degrees F for 25 minutes.

4. Serve right away.

Nutrition:

- Calories 246
- Fat 20.2
- Fiber 0.1
- Carbs 1.9
- Protein 14.5

19. Broccoli Dip

It's a reallyamazing combination! Try it!

Preparation time: 10 minutes

Cooking time: 30 minutes Servings: 8

Ingredients:

- 1 cup heavycream
- 1 pound broccoliflorets
- 2 springonions, chopped
- ¾ cup creamcheese
- ½ teaspoon chili powder
- Salt and black pepper to the taste
- 1 tablespoonchives, chopped

Directions:

1. In a pot, combine the creamwith the broccoli and the otheringredientsexceptthechives, stir, bring

to a simmer over medium heat and cook for 30 minutes.

2. Blend using an immersion blender, divideinto bowls, sprinkle the chives on topand serve cold.

Nutrition:

- Calories 149
- Fat 13.4
- Fiber 1.6
- Carbs 5.2
- Protein 3.6

20. Pesto Dip

It's one of the mosttastyketo snacks ever!

Preparation 5 minutes Cooking 0 minutes Servings: 8

Ingredients:

- 2 cups basil 1 cup parmesan, grated
- 1 tablespoon pine nuts, toasted
- 2 tablespoons olive oil garlicclove, minced
- A pinch of cayenne pepper

Directions:

1. In a blender, combine the basilwith the otheringredients, pulse well,

Nutrition:

- Calories 73 Fat 6.5 Fiber 0.2 Carbs 0.8 Protein 3.7

21. Zucchini Muffins

You can eventakethis snack at the office!

Preparation time: 10 minutes

Cooking time: 20 minutes

Servings: 6

Ingredients:

- ¼ cup coconutoil, melted
- 2 zucchinis, grated ¼ cup coconutflour
- ½ teaspoonnutmeg, ground
- ½ teaspoonbaking soda
- 2 eggs, whisked ½ teaspoonbakingpowder
- A pinch of salt

Directions:

1. In a bowl, combine the zucchinis with the oil and the otheringredients and stirreallywell.

2. Spoonthisinto a greased muffin pan, introduce in the oven at 370 degrees F andbake for 20 minutes.
3. Leave muffins to cool down and serve them as a snack.

Nutrition:

- Calories 131
- Fat 11.2
- Fiber 2.8
- Carbs 5.9
- Protein 3.3

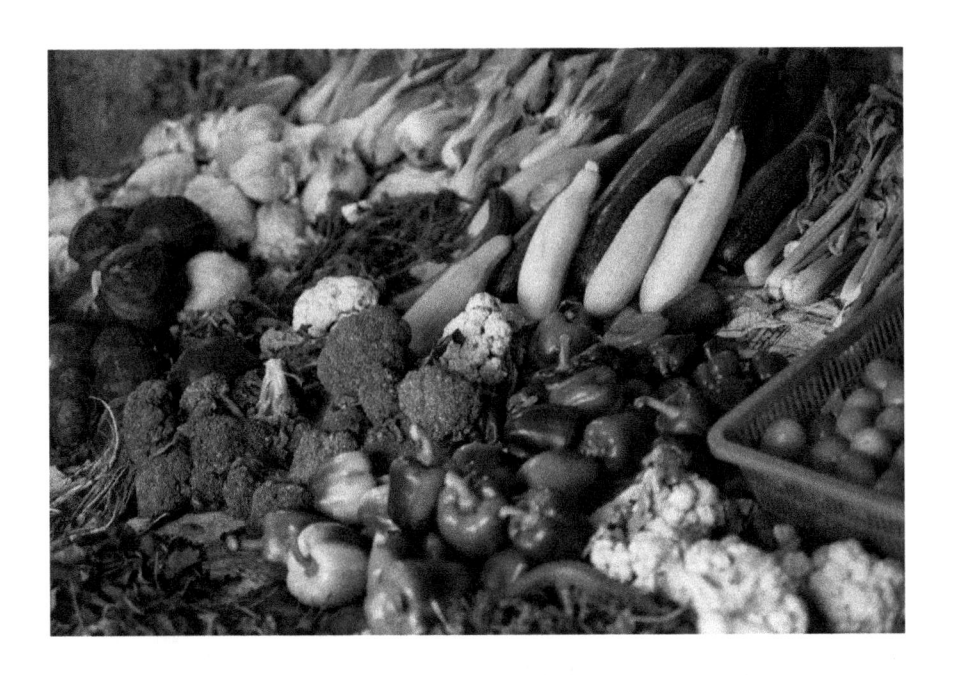

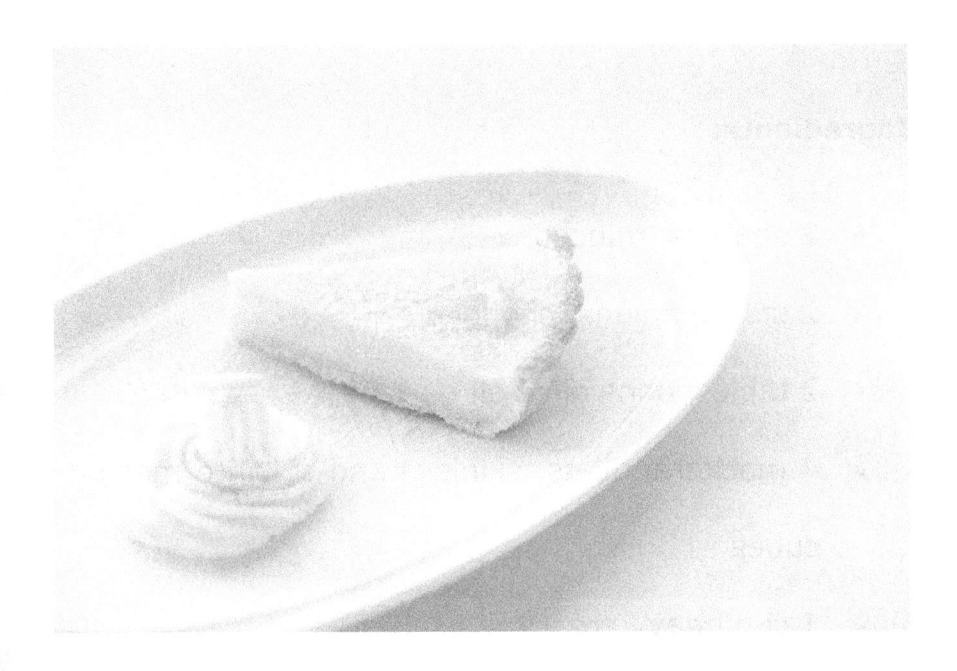

Ketogenic Diet For Beginners

KETOGENIC FISH AND SEAFOOD RECIPES

22.   Creamy Mackerel

This is really creamy and rich!

Preparation time: 10 minutes

Cooking time: 20 minutes

Servings: 4

Ingredients:

- 2 shallots, minced
- 2 spring onions, chopped
- 2 tablespoons olive oil
- 4 mackerel fillets, skinless and cut into medium cubes
- 1 cup heavy cream

- 1 teaspoon cumin, ground
- ½ teaspoon oregano, dried
- A pinch of salt and black pepper
- 2 tablespoons chives, chopped

Directions:

1. Heat up a pan with the oil over medium heat, add the spring onions and theshallots, stir and sauté for 5 minutes.
2. Add the fish and cook it for 4 minutes.
3. Add the rest of the ingredients, bring to a simmer, cook everything for 10minutes more, divide between plates and serve.

Nutrition:

- Calories 403 Fat 33.9
- Fiber 0.4 Carbs 2.7
- Protein 22

23. Lime Mackerel

It's an easyketodish for you to enjoytonight for dinner!

Preparation time: 10 minutes

Cooking time: 30 minutes

Servings: 4

Ingredients:

- 4 mackerelfillets, boneless
- 2 tablespoons lime juice
- 2 tablespoons olive oil
- A pinch of salt and black pepper
- ½ teaspoonsweet paprika

Directions:

1. Arrange the mackerel on a bakingsheetlinedwithparchmentpaper, add the oiland the otheringredients, rubgently, introduce

in the oven at 360 degrees F andbake for 30 minutes.

2. Divide the fishbetween plates and serve.

Nutrition:

- Calories 297
- Fat 22.7
- Fiber 0.2
- Carbs 2
- Protein 21.1

24. Turmeric Tilapia

This greatdishisperfect for a specialevening!

Preparation time: 10 minutes Cooking time: 12 minutes Servings: 4

Ingredients:

- 4 tilapia fillets, boneless
- 2 tablespoons olive oil
- 1 teaspoonturmericpowder
- A pinch of salt and black pepper
- 2 springonions, chopped
- ¼ teaspoonbasil, dried
- ¼ teaspoongarlicpowder
- 1 tablespoonparsley, chopped

Directions:

1. Heat up a pan with the oil over medium heat, add

the springonions and cookthem for 2minutes.

2. Add the fish, turmeric and the otheringredients, cook for 5 minutes on eachside, dividebetween plates and serve.

Nutrition:

- Calories 205
- Fat 8.6
- Fiber 0.4
- Carbs 1.1
- Protein 31.8

25. Walnut Salmon Mix

You just have to try this wonderful combination!

Preparation time: 10 minutes

Cooking time: 14 minutes

Servings: 4

Ingredients:

- 4 salmon fillets, boneless
- 2 tablespoons avocado oil
- A pinch of salt and black pepper
- 1 tablespoon lime juice 2 shallots, chopped
- 2 tablespoons walnuts, chopped
- 2 tablespoons parsley, chopped

Directions:

1. Heat up a pan with the oil over medium high heat, add the shallots, stir and sautéfor 2

minutes.

2. Add the fish and the other ingredients, cook for 6 minutes on each side, dividebetween plates and serve.

Nutrition:

- Calories 276
- Fat 14.2
- Fiber 0.7
- Carbs 2.7
- Protein 35.8

26. Chives Trout

The fish is so rich and flavored!

Preparation time: 10 minutes

Cooking time: 12 minutes

Servings: 4

Ingredients:

- 4 trout fillets, boneless
- 2 shallots, chopped
- A pinch of salt and black pepper
- 3 tablespoons chives, chopped
- 2 tablespoons avocado oil
- 2 teaspoons lime juice

Directions:

1. Heat up a pan with the oil over medium heat, add the shallots and sauté them for2 minutes.

2. Add the fish and the rest of the ingredients, cook for 5 minutes on each side, divide between plate sand serve.

Nutrition:

- Calories 320
- Fat 12
- Fiber 1
- Carbs 2
- Protein 24

27. Salmon and Tomatoes

Preparation 10 minutes Cooking 25 Servings: 4

Ingredients:

- 2 tablespoons avocado oil 4 salmon fillets, boneless 1 cup cherry tomatoes, halved
- 2 spring onions, chopped ½ cup chicken stock

Directions:

1. In a roasting pan, combine the fish with the oil and the other ingredients, introduce in the oven at 400 degrees F and bake for 25 minutes.
2. Divide between plates and serve.

Nutrition:

- Calories 200 Fat 12 Fiber 0 Carbs 3
- Protein 21

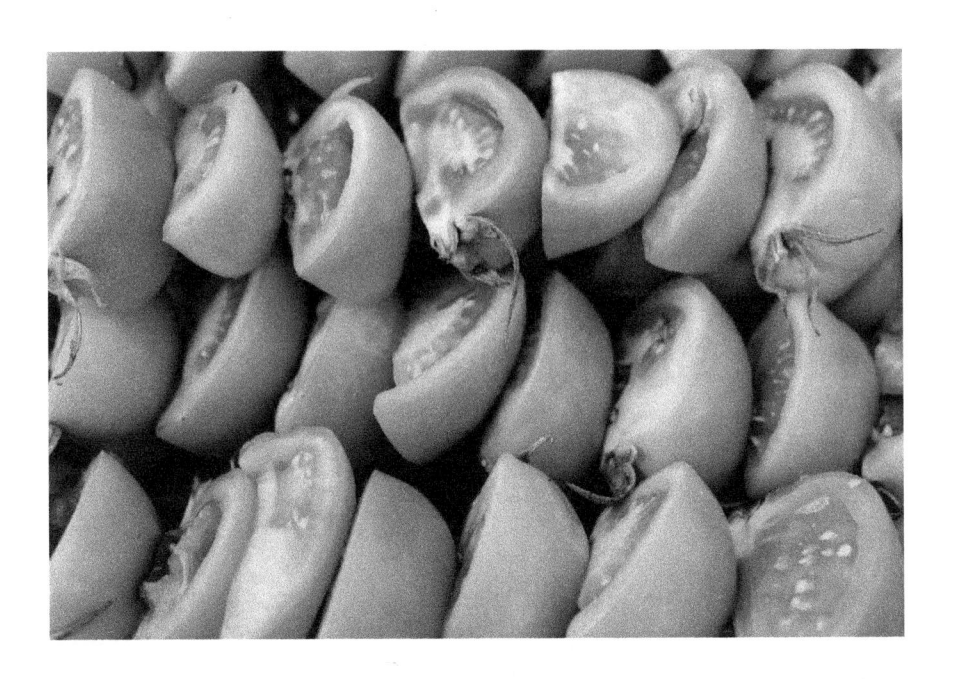

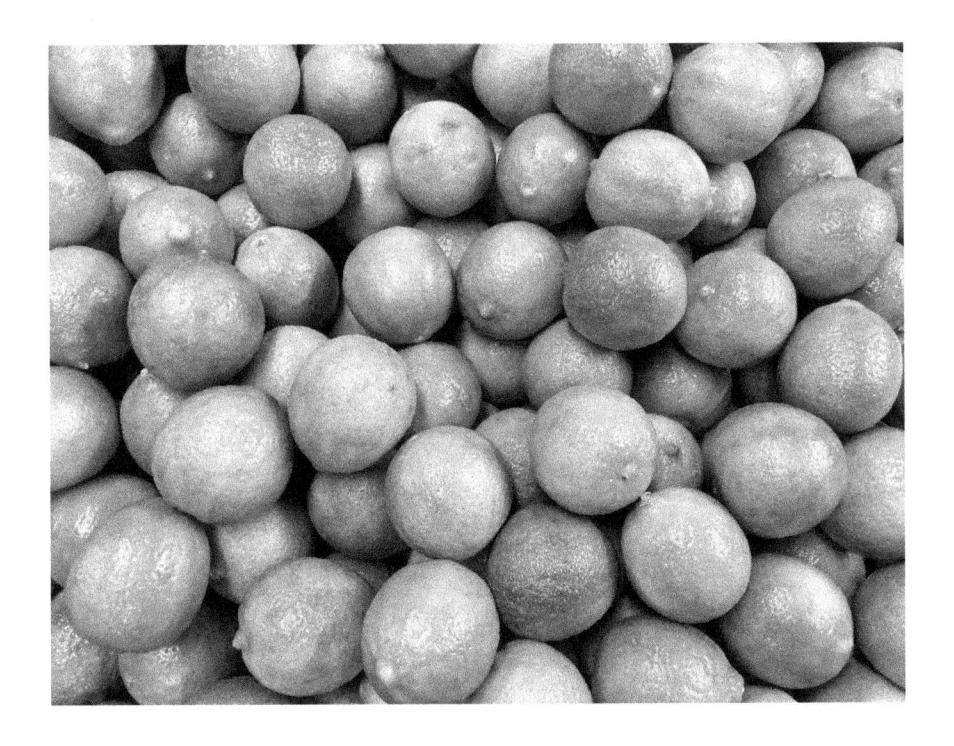

KETOGENIC POULTRY RECIPES

28. Ghee Chicken Mix

This is perfect for a friendly meal!

Preparation time: 10 minutes

Cooking time: 20 minutes

Servings: 4

Ingredients:

- 2 tablespoons garlic powder
- 2 chicken breasts, skinless boneless and sliced
- Salt and black pepper to the taste
- ½ cup ghee, melted
- ½ cup chicken stock
- 1 tablespoon cilantro, chopped

Directions:

1. Heat up a pan with the ghee over medium heat, add the chicken and cook for 5minutes on each side.
2. Add the rest of the ingredients, cook for 10 minutes more, divide between platesand serve.

Nutrition:

- Calories 439
- Fat 33.4
- Fiber 0.4
- Carbs 3.2
- Protein 31.3

29. Paprika Chicken Wings

It's so fresh and delicious!

Preparation time: 10 minutes Cooking time: 20 minutes Servings: 4

Ingredients:

- 1 pound chicken wings
- 1 tablespoon cumin, ground
- 1 teaspoon coriander, ground
- 1 tablespoon sweet paprika
- A pinch of salt and black pepper
- 1 tablespoon lime juice
- 2 tablespoons olive oil

Directions:

1. In a bowl, mix the chicken wings with the cumin and the other ingredients, toss, spread them on a

baking sheet lined with parchment paper and cook at 420degrees F for 20 minutes.

2. Divide between plates and serve.

Nutrition:

- Calories 286
- Fat 16
- Fiber 0.8
- Carbs 1.6
- Protein 33.3

30. Chicken and Capers

Hurry up and make this dish today!

Preparation time: 10 minutes

Cooking time: 15 minutes

Servings: 4

Ingredients:

- 1 pound chicken breast, skinless, boneless and sliced 1 tablespoon olive oil
- 1 tablespoons capers, drained
- 1 cup tomato passata
- A pinch of salt and black pepper
- 1 tablespoon parsley, chopped

Directions:

1. Heat up a pan with the oil over medium heat, add the chicken and cook for 4minutes on each side.

2. Add the rest of the ingredients, cook for 8 minutes more, divide between platesand serve.

Nutrition:

- Calories 166
- Fat 6.4
- Fiber 0.6
- Carbs 1.2
- Protein 24.6

31. Cilantro Wings

You will have these done in no time!

Preparation time: 10 minutes

Cooking time: 20 minutes

Servings: 4

Ingredients:

- 2 pounds chicken wings
- Juice of 1 lime
- 1 tablespoon olive oil
- ¼ cup cilantro, chopped
- 2 garlic cloves, minced
- A pinch of salt and black pepper

Directions:

1. In a bowl, mix the chicken wings with the lime juice and the other ingredients,toss and transfer

them to a roasting pan.

2. Introduce in the oven and cook at 390 degrees F for 20 minutes.

3. Divide the chicken wings between plates and serve with a side dish.

Nutrition:

- Calories 463
- Fat 20.3
- Fiber 0.1
- Carbs 0.6
- Protein 65.7

32. Baked Turkey Mix

It's a very simple keto chicken recipe!

Preparation time: 10 minutes

Cooking time: 30 minutes

Servings: 4

Ingredients:

- 1 big turkey breast, skinless, boneless and sliced

    3 green onions, chopped

- ½ cup tomato passata
- 1 tablespoon avocado oil
- 1 cup green olives, pitted and halved
- 2 tablespoons parmesan, grated

Directions:

1. Grease a baking dish with the oil, arrange the turkey slices inside, add the onionsand the other ingredients except the parmesan and toss.
2. Sprinkle the parmesan on top, introduce the dish in the oven and bake at 390degrees F for 30 minutes.
3. Divide the mix between plates and serve.

Nutrition:

- Calories 450
- Fat 24
- Fiber 0
- Carbs 3
- Protein 60

33. Turkey and Artichokes Mix

This is an Italian style keto dish we really appreciate!

Preparation time: 10 minutes

Cooking time: 25 minutes

Servings: 4

Ingredients:

- 2 tablespoons olive oil
- 1 red onion, chopped
- 1 cup chicken stock
- 1 big turkey breast, skinless, boneless and sliced
- 2 artichokes, trimmed and quartered
- 4 garlic cloves, minced
- A pinch of salt and black pepper
- ½ teaspoon red chili flakes
- 1 tablespoon cilantro, chopped

Directions:

1. Heat up a pan with the oil over medium heat, add the turkey and cook for 5minutes.
2. Add the onion and the other ingredients, cook everything over medium heat for20 minutes more, divide between plates and serve.

Nutrition:

- Calories 400
- Fat 20
- Fiber 1
- Carbs 2
- Protein 7

KETOGENIC MEAT RECIPES

34. Pork and Tomatoes

This pork dish will surprise you for sure!

Preparation time: 10 minutes

Cooking time: 45 minutes

Servings: 4

Ingredients:

- 2 tablespoons olive oil
- 1 pound pork loin, cubed
- 2 cups cherry tomatoes, halved
- 2 shallots, chopped
- 1 tablespoon lime juice
- 1 cup beef stock
- 1 teaspoon sweet paprika
- 1 teaspoon cumin, ground

- 1 tablespoon cilantro, chopped
- A pinch of salt and black pepper

Directions:

1. Heat up a pan with the oil over medium heat, add the meat and shallots andbrown for 5 minutes.
2. Add the rest of the ingredients, toss, introduce in the oven and bake at 390degrees F for 40 minutes.
3. Divide everything between plates and serve.

Nutrition:

- Calories 361
- Fat 23.3
- Fiber 1.4
- Carbs 5
- Protein 32

35. Garlic Pork and Zucchinis

Try this keto dish really soon!

Preparation time: 10 minutes

Cooking time: 35 minutes

Servings: 4

Ingredients:

- 2 tablespoons avocado oil
- 2 spring onions, chopped
- 1 pound pork stew meat, cubed
- 1 zucchini, cubed
- 3 garlic cloves, minced
- 1 cup tomato passata
- 1 cup cilantro, chopped
- A pinch of salt and black pepper
- 1 tablespoon oregano, chopped

Directions:

1. Heat up a pan with the oil over medium heat, add the garlic and the springonions, stir and sauté for 2 minutes.
2. Add the meat and brown for 5 minutes more.
3. Add the rest of the ingredients, toss, bring to a simmer and cook over mediumheat for 20 minutes more.
4. Divide everything into bowls and serve.

Nutrition:

- Calories 274
- Fat 12.1
- Fiber 2.2
- Carbs 5.2
- Protein 34.9

36. Balsamic Pork Chops

These pork chops are all you need to end this day!

Preparation time: 10 minutes

Cooking time: 20 minutes

Servings: 4

Ingredients:

- 4 pork chops 2 tablespoons olive oil
- 3 garlic cloves, minced
- 1 red onion, chopped
- 1 teaspoon nutmeg, ground
- 1 tablespoon balsamic vinegar
- 1 tablespoon rosemary, chopped

Directions:

1. Heat up a pan with the oil over medium heat, add the garlic and the pork chopsand brown for 3

minutes on each side.

2. Add the onion, and cook for 4 minutes more.

3. Add the rest of the ingredients, toss, cook over medium heat for 10 minutesmore, divide between plates and serve with a side salad.

Nutrition:

- Calories 337
- Fat 27.3
- Fiber 1.1
- Carbs 4.1
- Protein 18.5

37. Rosemary Pork

You must pay attention and learn how to make this tasty keto dish!

Preparation time: 10 minutes Cooking time: 30 minutes Servings: 4

Ingredients:

- 1 pound pork stew meat, roughly cubed
- 1 tablespoon olive oil
- 2 shallots, chopped
- 1 tablespoon rosemary, chopped
- 1 cup beef stock
- 1 teaspoon sweet paprika
- A pinch of salt and black pepper

Directions:

1. Heat up a pan with the oil over medium heat, add

the shallots and the meat and brown for 5minutes.

2. Add the rosemary and the other ingredients, toss, bring to a simmer and cook over medium heatfor 25 minutes more.

3. Divide the mix between plates and serve.

Nutrition:

- calories 279
- fat 14.8
- fiber 0.6
- carbs 0.9
- protein 34

KETOGENIC VEGETABLE RECIPES

38. Broccoli Cream

This issotextured and delicious!

Preparation time: 10 minutes

Cooking time: 20 minutes

Servings: 4

Ingredients:

- 1 pound broccoliflorets
- 4 cups vegetable stock
- 2 shallots, chopped
- 1 teaspoon chili powder
- A pinch of salt and black pepper
- 2 garliccloves, minced

- 2 tablespoons olive oil, chopped
- 1 tablespoondill, chopped

Directions:

1. Heat up a pot with the oil over medium high heat, add the shallots and the garlic and sauté for 2minutes.
2. Add the broccoli and the otheringredients, bring to a simmer and cook over medium heat for 18minutes.
3. Blend the mix using an immersion blender, divide the creaminto bowls and serve.

Nutrition:

- Calories 111 Fat 8
- Fiber 3.3
- Carbs 10.2
- Protein 3.7

39. Baked Broccoli

Preparation 10 Cooking 20 minutes Servings: 4

Ingredients:

- 2 garlic cloves, minced 2 tablespoons olive oil
- 1 pound broccoli florets ½ teaspoon nutmeg, ground ½ teaspoons rosemary, dried A pinch of salt and black pepper

Directions:

1. In a roasting pan, combine the broccoli with the garlic and the other ingredients, toss and bake at 400 degrees F for 20 minutes. Divide the mix between plates and serve.

Nutrition:

- Calories 150 Fat 4.1 Fiber 1 Carbs 3.2 Protein 2

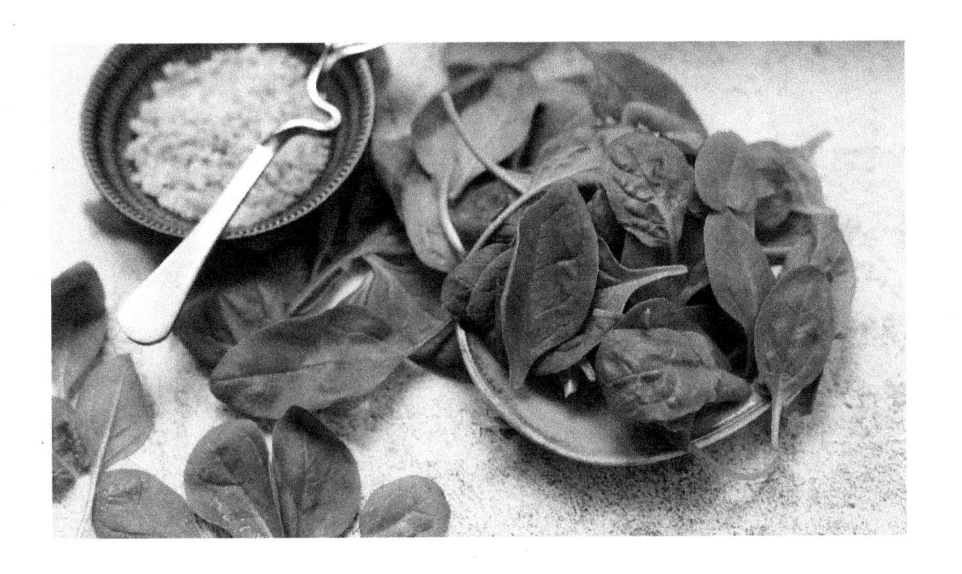

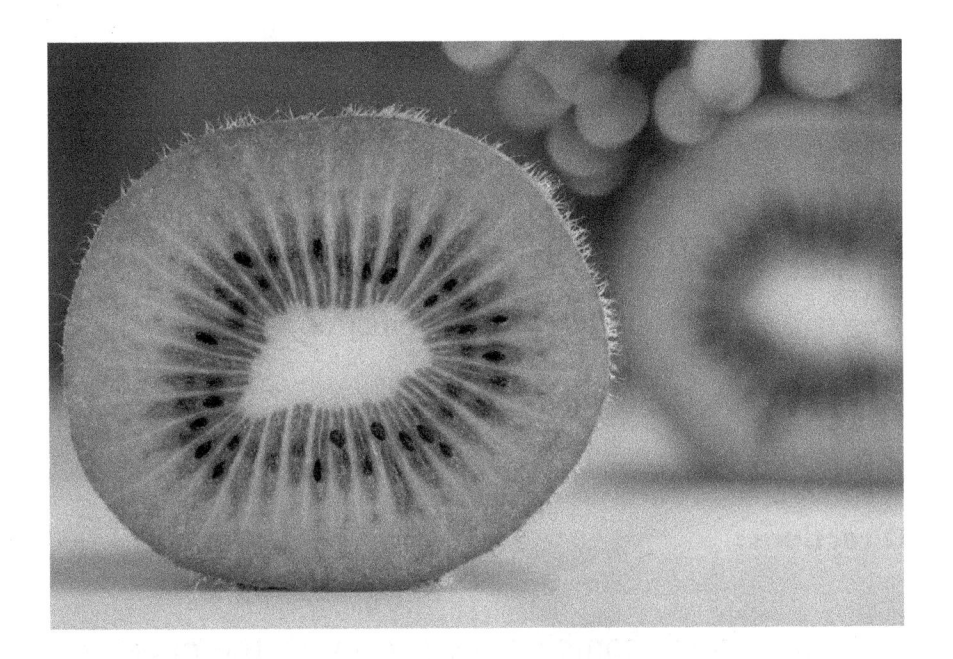

KETOGENIC DESSERT RECIPES

40. Chocolate Pudding

Theseissowonderful and delicious!

Preparation 10 minutes Cooking 20 min Servings: 4

Ingredients:

- 2 tablespoonscocoapowder
- 2 tablespoons ghee, melted
- 2/3 cup heavycream 2 tablespoonsswerve
- ¼ teaspoonvanillaextract

Directions:

1. In a bowl, combine the cocoawith the ghee and the otheringredients whisk well and divide into4

ramekins.

2. Bake at 350 degrees F for 20 minutes and serve warm.

Nutrition:

- Calories 134
- Fat 14.1
- Fiber 0.8
- Carbs 3.1
- Protein 0.9